HERBAL TINCTURES FOR WOMEN

24-Tincture Recipes for Women Health and Wellness

TABLE OF CONTENT

INTRODUCTION

Inspiration and life experience are the driving forces behind any successful undertaking. As a woman who has dealt with hormonal imbalances, menstruation abnormalities, and mood swings, I've been on a mission to find natural and holistic ways to improve my health.

Since I was unhappy with the standard medical approach, which focused more on treating symptoms, I decided to research herbal therapy and its possible advantages.

I investigated the wonderful medicinal characteristics of many plants and the potential of herbal tinctures in supporting women's health through thorough research and talks with herbalists and healthcare specialists.

After seeing the positive outcomes myself, I felt compelled to help other women by providing them with information about natural alternatives to traditional treatments.

I set out to write a book that combines scientific insights, practical assistance, and personal anecdotes because I wanted to make a difference in the field of women's health advocacy and because of my own experiences in this area.

This book seeks to remove the mystery surrounding herbal tinctures by providing a thorough reference for women to use in making health care decisions.

Herbal tinctures may be helpful for a variety of women's health issues, and this book investigates their possible advantages based on ancient wisdom, scientific research, and my own personal path.

It offers advice on how to choose, prepare, and properly utilize herbal tinctures for a variety of female health concerns, including those related to menstruation and hormone imbalances, reproductive health, menopause, and beyond.

My goal in writing about my experiences is to encourage and enable other women to take charge of their health by tapping into the healing potential of herbs and other natural remedies.

A woman's path of self-discovery and acceptance of natural solutions that nourish her body, mind, and spirit can be found in these pages.

CHAPTER ONE

Many health disorders affect both men and women, but there are also some issues that just affect women. It can be inspiring to learn about the most frequent women's health issues and how they evolve during a woman's lifetime. Moreover, the key to avoiding illness, maintaining good health, and thriving is learning about your own individual requirements in this area.

Women's health issues are not uniform; they differ by age, heredity, and lifestyle. While alcohol misuse, heart disease, mental health concerns, osteoarthritis, STIs, stress, stroke, and urinary tract health can all affect both men and women, they tend to have a greater impact on women.

Many different aspects of a woman's physical and mental health including those that are specific to her contribute to her total well-being.

Herbal tinctures are a popular natural remedy that have been used by women for centuries to treat a variety of health issues.

Plant and botanical-based tinctures, sometimes known as herbal remedies, have been used for their possible therapeutic effects on women's health.

Female Health Issues

Diseases like heart disease, stroke, and diabetes, which disproportionately affect women, can just as easily strike men. However, there are illnesses that primarily affect females. Diseases of the uterus, ovaries, fallopian tubes, and vagina are included here.

Cysts, fibroids, and malignancies are all possible in these organs. Due to the proximity of these organs to the digestive tract. Women are more likely to experience a variety of gastrointestinal problems. Some examples are IBS, constipation, IBD (including Crohn's disease and ulcerative colitis), gallstones, autoimmune liver disease, celiac disease, and dysfunction of the pelvic floor.

Some mental health issues are also more prevalent among women than men.

Depression and anxiety are more common in women than in men, and suicide is the second highest cause of death for women under the age of 60. In addition, women are disproportionately affected by domestic violence and sexual assault.

PMS (Premenstrual syndrome)

The symptoms of premenstrual syndrome (PMS) persist year after year for many women. In the last two weeks before menstruation, 40% of women experience premenstrual syndrome. Breast tenderness, acne, cramps, bloating, cravings, migraines, depression, anxiety, fatigue, and inability to fall or stay asleep are just a few of the many symptoms.

There are things you may do to alleviate the discomfort and mental drain of PMS. A carb-rich diet, high in grains and vegetables, is what you need. You should also get at least 30 minutes of exercise on three out of seven days.

It's also a good idea to supplement your diet with essential nutrients like calcium, magnesium, and vitamin B6.

Reproductive Health

In addition to PMS, sexual and reproductive health issues are particularly prevalent among women. Reproductive health issues account for a third of the issues experienced by women aged 15 to 44.

Reproductive health problems can be avoided by practicing safe sexual behavior. Anxiety, despair, and other mental health disorders are all potential outcomes of struggling with your reproductive health.

The Heart and Cardiovascular Disease

Many people have no warning signs of heart disease until it's too late. Among U.S. women, it is the leading cause of death. The risk of developing heart disease increases with the presence of risk factors such as hypertension, high cholesterol, diabetes, obesity, menopause, and a sedentary lifestyle.

The fact that many people don't get checked for cardiac problems contributes to the problem's lethality.

The good news is that you can take preventative measures against cardiovascular disease.

Each one has a positive side, though, in that it can help you live longer and healthier. The risk of cardiovascular disease can be lowered by engaging in regular physical activity, eating healthily, not smoking, and managing stress.

Cancers of the Breast and Cervix

Once a woman reaches maturity, she should start getting screened for cancer. Two of the most common cancers in women are the breast and the cervix. Cancer survival rates improve with earlier diagnosis. Cancer risk can be reduced through various lifestyle choices, but it cannot be completely avoided. Not finding out you have cancer until it has progressed is the leading cause of mortality from the disease.

The greatest way to detect breast and cervical cancer early is through annual screening.

Arthritis and Bone Fracture

The risk of developing osteoporosis or arthritis increases with age, particularly for women. Breaks and fractures are more likely to occur in people with osteoporosis since the condition weakens the bones.

However, arthritis attacks the joints, leading to severe inflammation in the area. Women of a certain age are disproportionately affected by these unpleasant disorders. Early screening and diagnosis of arthritis is the most effective method of preventing the disease. Exercise regularly, eat a diet rich in vitamin D and calcium, and supplement as needed to reduce your risk of developing osteoarthritis.

Wellness in Pregnancy

You should start protecting your prenatal health as soon as possible, whether or not you're pregnant. Having children is a physically demanding and taxing endeavor.

Prenatal health can be improved in several ways, including through the consumption of vegetables, calcium, and iron. Preparing your body for weight loss after giving birth can be aided by engaging in regular physical activity.

Beginning a folic acid supplement at least once daily at least three months before to a planned pregnancy is recommended.

Your unborn child's risk of developing neural tube abnormalities will be lowered as a result of this. If you want the finest advise and the most support, talk to doctors and the ladies in your life.

Transmission of HIV and Other STDs

Some of the most dangerous sexually transmitted diseases are HIV, gonorrhea, syphilis, and chlamydia. The best method to avoid contracting these diseases is to practice safe sexual behavior and wear protective gear. Hundreds of thousands of stillbirths and tens of thousands of newborn deaths can be attributed to untreated syphilis.

Disabilities in Mental Health

Women of all ages now seem to be more affected than ever by mental health issues. Depression, extreme anxiety, and a loss of hope are all possible outcomes of dealing with the rigors of daily life on top of the worry of uncertainty.

Suicide has surpassed automobile accidents as the biggest cause of mortality for women under the age of 60, and women are more likely than males to encounter mental health issues.

Seek professional help if you experience any of the symptoms of anxiety or depression. Reducing your stress levels is an important first step, but you may also benefit from counseling to restore your emotional health and well-being.

Disorders of Sleep and Insomnia

There has been a rise in the prevalence of sleep disorders including insomnia, particularly amongst women. Having a stressful lifestyle and eating poorly are common causes.

Anxiety and other mental problems are frequently accompanied by sleep disturbances. One of the most crucial parts of maintaining a healthy lifestyle is sleeping well every night. The most effective treatments for insomnia and other sleep disorders are medication and the development of a consistent sleep regimen.

Knowing what to expect as you age might help you maintain your health and catch problems early on. A woman's health can decline at any point in her life. Between the ages of 15 and 44, many people experience problems with their sexual and reproductive health. However, major diseases like cancer and heart disease tend to manifest in middle age.

At Teen

Fortunately, adolescent girls rarely have serious health issues. Menstruation is the primary source of distress for young women. Endometriosis and dysmenorrhea (painful menstrual cycles) are two conditions that can affect teenage girls.

<u>At 20s</u>

Women's sexual health and the prevention of sexually transmitted infections rise to the forefront when they enter their twenties. Fertility can be negatively impacted by health problems that manifest in one's twenties, such as sexually transmitted diseases and pelvic inflammatory disease. Some others are:

<u>Melanoma</u>

The risk of developing malignant melanoma, the worst form of skin cancer, increases with age. However, among young adults, especially women, it is one of the most often diagnosed cancers. Intense sun exposure in your twenties has been linked to an increased risk of melanoma in later life. Early prevention is key, so try to limit your time in the sun and always use sunscreen. You should also visit a dermatologist regularly for checkups and look for any strange spots on your skin.

Even though youth smoking rates have gone down, it is still the greatest cause of preventable mortality in the United States. The effects of drinking and smoking in one's twenties might be felt decades later. If you quit smoking before you are 30, you can reduce your risk of dying from lung cancer by more than 90 percent. Consistent heavy drinking in one's twenties has also been linked to an increased risk of cancer and liver disease.

At 30s

Fertility issues and postpartum difficulties are common concerns for women in their 30s. Gestational diabetes and preeclampsia are two pregnancy- and childbirth-related disorders that, if left untreated, can cause serious complications or even death.

Fertility often declines in one's 30s, making pregnancy more of a challenge. Pregnancy-related health issues and miscarriage are more common in women aged 35 and over.

Preeclampsia (chronic high blood pressure), Gestational Diabetes, and Hypertension in Pregnancy Chronic hypertension, Stress, worry, and melancholy, Infections

Our metabolic rate inevitably decreases with aging. Weight gain or difficulty losing weight is a common problem for women in their 30s. Putting on too much weight is not usually a symptom of a health concern, but it can worsen conditions including diabetes, high blood pressure, and infertility.

At 40s

Women's health after 40 focuses on perimenopause, a time when a woman's ovaries produce fewer eggs, her progesterone and estrogen levels drop, and her menstrual cycles become irregular. Menopause occurs after a woman has gone 12 months without having her period, therefore perimenopause can continue anywhere from two to ten years. Menstrual abnormalities, hot flashes, vaginal dryness, disturbed sleep, pain with intercourse, infertility, weight gain, and irritability are all caused by a lack of ovarian hormones.

It's possible that conditions like diabetes, hypertension, heart disease, obesity, and infertility might rise to the forefront during this time as well.

Osteoporosis is a disease that weakens bones, and it may be more common among women in their forties. After the age of 40, nearly all women will enter menopause. Although menopause itself is not a medical illness, the physiological changes that accompany it are.

Less estrogen is produced by the ovaries after menopause. The chance of developing certain diseases and disorders increases in women whose estrogen levels are low. Cholesterol accumulation and an increased risk of heart disease have both been linked to inadequate estrogen levels. In addition, it may increase or decrease your vulnerability to lead poisoning, urinary incontinence, and osteoporosis.

<u>After the age of 50</u>

Many gynecological symptoms, such as urine incontinence, vaginal atrophy and dryness, and discomfort with intercourse (dyspareunia), might emerge at this age because of menopause. Diseases including cancer, osteoporosis, and diabetes are also a concern.

CHAPTER TWO

Use of Herbs as a Woman

Most modern women in developed nations rely on medications and allopathic medicine to address and maintain reproductive health. While there is a place for traditional medicine, often the gentlest and most harmonic solutions can be found in nature.

Most, if not all, traditional medical practices include the use of herbs. It's predicated on the idea that people and the natural world are inseparable, and that the remedies for their problems might be right in their own backyards. The world of plants is the entry point to the possibilities of self-healing and bodily agency, and it may be easier to access than conventional medical practices.

It's vital to trust your instincts when you're initially learning to utilize herbalism to treat your health problems, as the process can seem overwhelming if you're unfamiliar with it. Finding a treatment that helps can take time, but there are several options that have been shown to be effective.

Knowing the various routes of ingestion for various herbs is essential before going into which ones might be helpful for you.

Teas: Something we're all familiar with. What many people don't realize is that this heartwarming ritual is an integral part of herbalism. Making tea from fresh or dried herbs either prepared, or making your own mixtures makes for a gentle introduction into herbalism.

Tinctures: Concentrated herbal extractions typically preserved in alcohol.

Capsules: Powdered herbs packed into tiny gel capsules. You can even make your own by using a capsule kit.

Essential Oils: With their growing popularity, essential oils are becoming a star player in many people's home apothecaries. Clary sage, ylang, ylang, and lavender diluted in a carrier oil and applied to abdomen can help ease menstrual cramps.

Salves: Many topical treatments are infused with herbs for their medicinal value, and comforting scents.

Black cohosh

Helps in easing menstrual cramps as well as hot flashes during menopause.

Calendula

Also known as Marigold, is known for its anti-inflammatory and wound-healing abilities. Calendula boosts the immune system and detoxifies the body. It can also help relieve breast tenderness and soothe cramps.

Chamomile buds

Many of us are familiar with this blissful bud for its calming effects. The glycine in chamomile helps relieve muscle contractions, AKA cramps, by relaxing blood vessels.

Dong Quai

A power play in Chinese medicine. It is believed to have an adaptogenic effect on the female hormonal system, helping to balance symptoms of PMS and menopause.

Fennel seeds

Commonly used for gas, bloating and digestive issues, fennel also packs a punch when used for periods pains.

Hibiscus

Filled with antioxidants and nutrients, hibiscus protects the liver, while the flavonoids can help calm the nervous system, boosting your mood. It can also help regulate your cycle by stimulating blood flow in the pelvic area

Lady's Mantle

This soothing herb calms PMS symptoms and even lighten a heavy flow, all while regulating your cycle.

Nettles

The high mineral content of this stinging "weed" can be easily found wild in many areas. Its benefits are neverending from detoxifying blood through the kidneys, cleansing the liver, and helping anemia thanks to its high iron content.

Oat Straw

Safe to take during all periods of the reproductive cycle, including while pregnant or nursing, oatstraw relieves stress and calms the body.

Red Raspberry Leaf

Helps to treat PMS symptoms like cramping and loose stools. It is known for its ability to tone and strengthen the uterus, regulating heavy and irregular periods, easing cramps and even helping in labor. Much of this is thanks to its high calcium and magnesium content. Mineral deficiency is a huge contributing factor when it comes to period pains.

Rose buds

Beautiful rose buds are popular in traditional Chinese medicine to relieve period cramping and treat hormonal conditions in women. Usually consumed in a relaxing tea, it helps to ease feelings of anxiety, stress and irritability.

St John's Wort

Mellows PMS symptoms, such as cravings, insomnia, headaches, negative emotions and fatigue.

Turmeric

This popular root is known for its anti-inflammatory and healing powers. The curcumin compound found in it can help to alleviate PMS symptoms.

Sage

Sage is an herb known for its strong herbal aroma and earthy flavor, it is often used medicinally and as an ornamental plant.

Phytoestrogens are plant derived non-steroidal oestrogens that are far milder than human derived oestrogen. Sage exerts mild phytoestrogenic properties, which could suggest why sage has been used as a remedy for menopausal symptoms, such as flushing, night sweats, heart palpitations muscle and joint pain, anxiety, depression, sleep disorders and sexual desire.

It is common for females to experience brain fog, and loss of memory during the peri-menopause and menopause.

Cranberry

The cranberry is a small hard, round, red fruit which can taste rather bitter and sour. Cranberries are native to North America and are often consumed in the form of a sauce or juice.

Urinary tract infections (UTI) are common in women, with many women experiencing more than one infection during their lifetime. A risk factor specific to women for being at a higher risk of developing a UTI is because a woman has a shorter urethra than a man does, this shortens the distance that the bacteria must travel to reach the bladder. Cranberries are well known for preventing UTIs, E. coli being the most common bacterial cause of UTIs.

Cranberries may help to minimize the visible signs of ageing, hyperpigmentation and loss of elasticity. Cranberries are a rich source of several vitamins and minerals, specifically vitamin C, a potent antioxidant.

Antioxidants help scavenge free radicals from the body cells and prevent or reduce damage that is caused by oxidation. Oxidative stress occurs when there is an imbalance between the production of free radicals and antioxidants in the body. It plays a major role in the ageing process. Oxidative stress can lead to chronic inflammation, and cause collagen fragmentation and inefficiency of collagen fibres and skin cell functions.

Saffron

Saffron is a spice which originates from a flower called crocus sativus, often known as the saffron crocus.

Saffron has a long history of use for improving mental health, including depression, anxiety and premenstrual syndrome. A number of possible mechanisms of action may explain the mental health benefits of saffron including, improvements in the action of the neurotransmitter serotonin, enhancement of brain functions such as memory and learning, antioxidant effects, and protecting the brain against the damaging effects of chronic stress.

Major depressive disorder (MDD) is a well-known mood disorder that can require long-term treatment. A number of clinical trials have suggested saffron as an alternative remedy to anti-depressant medication.

Shatavari

Shatavari is a species of asparagus that is native to India and the Himalayas. It is a general tonic and female reproductive tonic high in isoflavones.

Shatavari has been used in menopause as an antispasmodic, against menstrual cramps and as a uterine tonic, helping to regulate uterine function during different stages of the menstrual cycle.

CHAPTER THREE

Tincture Recipes for Women Health

1. Calming Chamomile Tincture

Preparation Time: 4-6 weeks

Ingredients

- Dried chamomile flowers

- Alcohol (such as vodka or brandy)

Directions

- Fill a jar halfway with dried chamomile flowers.

- Pour enough alcohol to completely cover the flowers.

- Close the jar tightly and let it sit for 4-6 weeks, shaking daily.

- Strain the tincture and store it in a dark glass bottle.

Dosage: Take 1-2 teaspoons, up to three times a day.

__Ailment__: Promotes relaxation, aids in sleep, soothes anxiety.

__Advice__: Avoid if allergic to chamomile or taking sedative medications.

__Side Effects__: May cause drowsiness in some individuals.

2. Hormone Balancing Tincture

Preparation Time: 4-6 weeks

Ingredients

- Vitex (Chaste tree berry)

- Dong quai root

- Black cohosh root

- Alcohol

Directions

- Combine equal parts of the herbs in a jar.

- Add enough alcohol to cover the herbs.

- Seal the jar and let it sit for 4-6 weeks, shaking daily.

- Strain the tincture and store it in a dark glass bottle.

__Dosage__: Take 1 teaspoon, twice daily.

__Ailment__: Regulates menstrual cycles, supports hormonal balance.

__Advice__: Not recommended during pregnancy or for individuals with hormone-sensitive conditions.

__Side Effects__: May cause digestive upset in some individuals.

3. Digestive Aid Tincture

Preparation Time: 4-6 weeks

Ingredients

- Peppermint leaves

- Ginger root

- Fennel seeds

- Alcohol

Directions

- Combine equal parts of the herbs in a jar.

- Add enough alcohol to cover the herbs.

- Seal the jar and let it sit for 4-6 weeks, shaking daily.

- Strain the tincture and store it in a dark glass bottle.

Dosage: Take 1-2 teaspoons, up to three times a day before meals.

Ailment: Relieves indigestion, bloating, and nausea.

Advice: Avoid if allergic to any of the herbs or taking anticoagulant medications.

Side Effects: May cause heartburn or allergic reactions in some individuals.

4. Immune Boosting Tincture

Preparation Time: 4-6 weeks

Ingredients

- Echinacea root

- Elderberry

- Astragalus root

- Alcohol

Directions

- Combine equal parts of the herbs in a jar.

- Add enough alcohol to cover the herbs.

- Seal the jar and let it sit for 4-6 weeks, shaking daily.

- Strain the tincture and store it in a dark glass bottle.

Dosage: Take 1 teaspoon, three times a day.

Ailment: Supports immune system function, helps prevent colds and flu.

__Advice__: Avoid if allergic to any of the herbs or have an autoimmune condition.

__Side Effects:__ Rare, but may cause allergic reactions in some individuals.

5. Sleep Support Tincture

Preparation Time: 4-6 weeks

Ingredients

- Valerian root

- Passionflower

- Hops

- Alcohol

Directions

- Combine equal parts of the herbs in a jar.

- Add enough alcohol to cover the herbs.

- Seal the jar and let it sit for 4-6 weeks, shaking daily.

- Strain the tincture and store it in a dark glass bottle.

__Dosage__: Take 1-2 teaspoons, 30 minutes before bedtime.

__Ailment__: Promotes restful sleep, relieves insomnia.

__Advice__: Avoid if pregnant, breastfeeding, or taking sedative medications.

__Side Effects__: May cause drowsiness or vivid dreams in some individuals.

6. Nerve Calming Tincture

Preparation Time: 4-6 weeks

Ingredients

- Skullcap

- Lemon balm

- California poppy

- Alcohol

Directions

- Combine equal parts of the herbs in a jar.

- Add enough alcohol to cover the herbs.

- Seal the jar and let it sits for 4-6 weeks, shaking daily.

- Strain the tincture and store it in a dark glass bottle.

**Dosage**: Take 1 teaspoon, up to three times a day.

**Ailment**: Soothes nervous tension, anxiety, and promotes relaxation.

**Advice**: Avoid if allergic to any of the herbs or taking sedative medications.

**Side Effects**: Rare, but may cause dizziness or drowsiness in some individuals.

7. Menstrual Cramp Relief Tincture

Preparation Time: 4-6 weeks

Ingredients

- Cramp bark

- Black haw

- Motherwort

- Alcohol

Directions

- Combine equal parts of the herbs in a jar.

- Add enough alcohol to cover the herbs.

- Seal the jar and let it sit for 4-6 weeks, shaking daily.

- Strain the tincture and store it in a dark glass bottle.

Dosage: Take 1 teaspoon, up to three times a day as needed during menstruation.

Ailment: Relieves menstrual cramps and muscle tension.

Advice: Avoid during pregnancy or if allergic to any of the herbs.

Side Effects: Rare, but may cause mild stomach upset in some individuals.

8. Urinary Tract Support Tincture

Preparation Time: 4-6 weeks

Ingredients

- Dandelion root

- Corn silk

- Uva ursi

- Alcohol

Directions

- Combine equal parts of the herbs in a jar.

- Add enough alcohol to cover the herbs.

- Seal the jar and let it sit for 4-6 weeks, shaking daily.

- Strain the tincture and store it in a dark glass bottle.

Dosage: Take 1 teaspoon, up to three times a day.

Ailment: Supports urinary tract health, relieves UTI symptoms.

Advice: Not recommended during pregnancy or for individuals with kidney disorders.

Side Effects: May cause mild stomach upset or allergic reactions in some individuals.

9. Allergy Relief Tincture

Preparation Time: 4-6 weeks

Ingredients

- Nettle leaf

- Eyebright

- Red clover

- Alcohol

Directions

- Combine equal parts of the herbs in a jar.

- Add enough alcohol to cover the herbs.

- Seal the jar and let it sit for 4-6 weeks, shaking daily.

- Strain the tincture and store it in a dark glass bottle.

Dosage: Take 1 teaspoon, up to three times a day.

Ailment: Reduces symptoms of seasonal allergies, such as sneezing and itchy eyes.

Advice: Avoid if allergic to any of the herbs or taking blood-thinning medications.

Side Effects: Rare, but may cause mild digestive upset or allergic reactions in some individuals.

10. Blood Cleansing Tincture

Preparation Time: 4-6 weeks

Ingredients

- Burdock root

- Red clover

- Yellow dock root

- Alcohol

Directions

- Combine equal parts of the herbs in a jar.

- Add enough alcohol to cover the herbs.

- Seal the jar and let it sit for 4-6 weeks, shaking daily.

- Strain the tincture and store it in a dark glass bottle.

Dosage: Take 1 teaspoon, up to three times a day.

Ailment: Supports liver function, detoxification, and overall blood health.

Advice: Not recommended during pregnancy or for individuals on blood-thinning medications.

Side Effects: May cause mild digestive upset in some individuals.

11.   Memory and Focus Tincture

Preparation Time: 4-6 weeks

Ingredients

- Ginkgo biloba

- Gotu kola

- Rosemary

- Alcohol

Directions

- Combine equal parts of the herbs in a jar.

- Add enough alcohol to cover the herbs.

- Seal the jar and let it sit for 4-6 weeks, shaking daily.

- Strain the tincture and store it in a dark glass bottle.

Dosage: Take 1 teaspoon, up to three times a day.

Ailment: Enhances memory, concentration, and cognitive function.

Advice: Avoid if taking blood-thinning medications or have a bleeding disorder.

Side Effects: Rare, but may cause headache or allergic reactions in some individuals.

12.   Energy Boosting Tincture

Preparation Time: 4-6 weeks

Ingredients

- Ginseng (Panax or Siberian)

- Ashwagandha root

- Licorice root

- Alcohol

Directions

- Combine equal parts of the herbs in a jar.

- Add enough alcohol to cover the herbs.

- Seal the jar and let it sit for 4-6 weeks, shaking daily.

- Strain the tincture and store it in a dark glass bottle.

**Dosage**: Take 1 teaspoon, up to three times a day.

**Ailment**: Increases energy levels, combats fatigue, and supports adrenal health.

**Advice**: Avoid if pregnant, breastfeeding, or have high blood pressure.

**Side Effects**: Rare, but may cause digestive upset or interact with certain medications.

13.   Joint Pain Relief Tincture

Preparation Time: 4-6 weeks

Ingredients

- Turmeric

- Devil's claw root

- White willow bark

- Alcohol

Directions

- Combine equal parts of the herbs in a jar.

- Add enough alcohol to cover the herbs.

- Seal the jar and let it sit for 4-6 weeks, shaking daily.

- Strain the tincture and store it in a dark glass bottle.

Dosage: Take 1 teaspoon, up to three times a day.

Ailment: Relieves joint pain, inflammation, and stiffness.

Advice: Not recommended for individuals with bleeding disorders or on anticoagulant medications.

Side Effects: May cause digestive upset or interact with certain medications.

14.   Heart Health Tincture

Preparation Time: 4-6 weeks

Ingredients

- Hawthorn berries

- Motherwort

- Garlic

- Alcohol

Directions

- Combine equal parts of the herbs in a jar.

- Add enough alcohol to cover the herbs.

- Seal the jar and let it sit for 4-6 weeks, shaking daily.

- Strain the tincture and store it in a dark glass bottle.

Dosage: Take 1 teaspoon, up to three times a day.

Ailment: Supports cardiovascular health, strengthens the heart, and regulates blood pressure.

Advice: Consult with a healthcare provider if taking heart medications or have a heart condition.

Side Effects: Rare, but may cause mild stomach upset or interact with certain medications.

15.   Hair and Scalp Tonic Tincture

Preparation Time: 4-6 weeks

Ingredients

- Horsetail

- Nettle leaf

- Rosemary

- Alcohol

Directions

- Combine equal parts of the herbs in a jar.

- Add enough alcohol to cover the herbs.

- Seal the jar and let it sit for 4-6 weeks, shaking daily.

- Strain the tincture and store it in a dark glass bottle.

Dosage: Apply topically by massaging a few drops into the scalp after washing the hair.

Ailment: Promotes hair growth, strengthens hair follicles, and improves scalp health.

__Advice__: Avoid if allergic to any of the herbs or have sensitive skin.

__Side Effects__: Rare, but may cause skin irritation in some individuals.

16.   Anxiety Relief Tincture

Preparation Time: 4-6 weeks

Ingredients

- Lemon balm

- Passionflower

- Lavender

- Alcohol

Directions

- Combine equal parts of the herbs in a jar.

- Add enough alcohol to cover the herbs.

- Seal the jar and let it sit for 4-6 weeks, shaking daily.

- Strain the tincture and store it in a dark glass bottle.

__Dosage__: Take 1 teaspoon, up to three times a day.

__Ailment__: Reduces anxiety, promotes relaxation, and calms the nervous system.

__Advice__: Avoid if pregnant, breastfeeding, or taking sedative medications.

__Side Effects__: Rare, but may cause mild stomach upset or drowsiness in some individuals.

17.   Skin Clearing Tincture

Preparation Time: 4-6 weeks

Ingredients

- Burdock root

- Dandelion root

- Oregon grape root

- Alcohol

Directions

- Combine equal parts of the herbs in a jar.

- Add enough alcohol to cover the herbs.

- Seal the jar and let it sit for 4-6 weeks, shaking daily.

- Strain the tincture and store it in a dark glass bottle.

Dosage: Take 1 teaspoon, up to three times a day.

Ailment: Clears acne and supports overall skin health.

Advice: Not recommended during pregnancy or breastfeeding.

Side Effects: May cause mild digestive upset in some individuals.

18.   Respiratory Support Tincture

Preparation Time: 4-6 weeks

Ingredients

- Mullein

- Marshmallow root

- Elecampane root

- Alcohol

- Combine equal parts of the herbs in a jar.

- Add enough alcohol to cover the herbs.

- Seal the jar and let it sit for 4-6 weeks, shaking daily.

- Strain the tincture and store it in a dark glass bottle.

Dosage: Take 1 teaspoon, up to three times a day.

Ailment: Relieves cough, congestion, and supports respiratory health.

Advice: Avoid if allergic to any of the herbs or have asthma.

Side Effects: Rare, but may cause mild stomach upset or allergic reactions in some individuals.

19.   Stress Relief Tincture

Ingredients

- Ashwagandha root

- Skullcap

- Lemon balm

- Alcohol

Directions

- Combine equal parts of the herbs in a jar.

- Add enough alcohol to cover the herbs.

- Seal the jar and let it sit for 4-6 weeks, shaking daily.

- Strain the tincture and store it in a dark glass bottle.

Dosage: Take 1 teaspoon, up to three times a day.

Ailment: Reduces stress, promotes relaxation, and supports adrenal health.

**Advice**: Avoid if pregnant, breastfeeding, or have low blood pressure.

**Side Effects**: Rare, but may cause digestive upset or interact with certain medications.

20.   Muscle Relaxation Tincture

Preparation Time: 4-6 weeks

Ingredients

- Kava root

- Valerian root

- Passionflower

- Alcohol

Directions

- Combine equal parts of the herbs in a jar.

- Add enough alcohol to cover the herbs.

- Seal the jar and let it sit for 4-6 weeks, shaking daily.

- Strain the tincture and store it in a dark glass bottle.

**Dosage**: Take 1 teaspoon, up to three times a day.

**Ailment**: Relieves muscle tension, spasms, and promotes relaxation.

**Advice**: Avoid if pregnant, breastfeeding, or taking sedative medications.

**Side Effects**: May cause drowsiness or interact with certain medications.

21.   Liver Detox Tincture

Preparation Time: 4-6 weeks

Ingredients

- Milk thistle

- Dandelion root

- Yellow dock root

- Alcohol

Directions

- Combine equal parts of the herbs in a jar.

- Add enough alcohol to cover the herbs.

- Seal the jar and let it sit for 4-6 weeks, shaking daily.

- Strain the tincture and store it in a dark glass bottle.

Dosage: Take 1 teaspoon, up to three times a day.

Ailment: Supports liver function, aids in detoxification, and promotes healthy digestion.

Advice: Avoid if allergic to any of the herbs or have gallbladder issues.

Side Effects: Rare, but may cause mild digestive upset in some individuals.

22.   Libido Boosting Tincture

Preparation Time: 4-6 weeks

Ingredients

- Damiana

- Maca root

- Tribulus terrestris (aphrodisiac)

- Alcohol

- Combine equal parts of the herbs in a jar.

- Add enough alcohol to cover the herbs.

- Seal the jar and let it sit for 4-6 weeks, shaking daily.

- Strain the tincture and store it in a dark glass bottle.

Dosage: Take 1 teaspoon, up to three times a day.

Ailment: Enhances libido, improves sexual vitality, and supports reproductive health.

Advice: Not recommended during pregnancy or for individuals with hormone-sensitive conditions.

Side Effects: Rare, but may cause mild digestive upset or interact with certain medications.

23. Antioxidant Powerhouse Tincture

Preparation Time: 4-6 weeks

Ingredients

- Green tea

- Hawthorn berries

- Bilberry

- Alcohol

Directions

- Combine equal parts of the herbs in a jar.

- Add enough alcohol to cover the herbs.

- Seal the jar and let it sit for 4-6 weeks, shaking daily.

- Strain the tincture and store it in a dark glass bottle.

Dosage: Take 1 teaspoon, up to three times a day.

**Ailment**: Provides powerful antioxidant support, protects against oxidative stress.

**Advice**: Avoid if allergic to any of the herbs or have caffeine sensitivity.

**Side Effects**: Rare, but may cause mild stomach upset or interact with certain medications.

24.   Mood-Enhancing Tincture

Preparation Time: 4-6 weeks

Ingredients

- St. John's wort

- Lemon balm

- Passionflower

- Alcohol

Directions

- Combine equal parts of the herbs in a jar.

- Add enough alcohol to cover the herbs.

- Seal the jar and let it sit for 4-6 weeks, shaking daily.

- Strain the tincture and store it in a dark glass bottle.

Dosage: Take 1 teaspoon, up to three times a day.

Ailment: Lifts mood, reduces symptoms of mild depression and anxiety.

Advice: Avoid if taking antidepressant medications or have bipolar disorder.

Side Effects: May cause photosensitivity or interact with certain medications.

CONCLUSION

Keep in mind that this book is not meant to replace the counsel of a physician. Please seek the advice of a licensed medical practitioner or herbalist if you have any medical questions or concerns, especially if you are using any drugs.

Keep asking questions, be receptive to new information, and trust your body's intuition as you move forward on your path. Try out various tinctures made from the many different herbs and botanicals out there to see which ones work best for you. Have faith in the restorative properties of nature and in your own capacity to provide for your own health and well-being.

It's important to keep in mind that reaching your full potential in terms of health demands tending to your entire being, not just your physical body. Take time for yourself, eat healthily, move your body frequently, and surround yourself with positive, encouraging people.

Now that we've reached the end of the book, I hope you'll incorporate the lessons you've learned into your everyday life. May it serve as a beacon that encourages you to make decisions that are best for your health and happiness. You have the ability to write your own health story, so go headfirst into the process of self-reflection and self-care.

I appreciate you coming along with me as I learn about herbal tinctures and their applications in the realm of women's health. Good health, happiness, and a strong bond with nature are my wishes for you on your journey. May you find strength in being a voice for your own health and a role model for those women who are interested in alternative medicine and wellness.

I hope you enjoy a life of harmony and vitality, and that your health always shines brightly.

With affection and appreciation,

RELINA VANGAR